KETO DIET

FOR WOMEN OVER 50

Find Out Why You Need to Start a Ketogenic Diet Right Now. A Complete Guide to Lose Weight and Speed Up Your Metabolism in Just a Few Days.

Gracelynn Rogers

TABLE OF CONTENTS

DINNER RECIPES 85

INTRODUCTION

The name "Keto" comes from the word "ketogenic" which refers to the metabolic state of ketosis that starts in the body when carbohydrate intake is suddenly reduced and replaced with healthy fats. Most people start a ketogenic diet to lose weight, not just in water weight but in abdominal and other stored fat. It resembles the Atkins and other low-carb diets.

The primary guideline is to drastically reduce your consumption of carbohydrates and replace them with healthy fats. This dramatic reduction in carbohydrates helps your body enter a metabolic state called ketosis in which your body burns fat for fuel rather than glucose.

The average person eats foods loaded in carbohydrates; the liver then converts glucose. Your body creates insulin in order to move the glucose into the bloodstream, which distributes it throughout your body and brain. The body's primary source of energy is glucose whenever carbohydrates are present in the body. Your body will always use glucose over fat or any other energy source.

The keto diet is focused on not using glucose as your energy source but instead fat. Once your body enters ketosis, your body becomes effective at burning fat, losing weight, and overall improving health. It also converts fat into ketones inside your liver, which can supply energy for the brain. The ketogenic diet can cause also cause a massive reduction in blood sugar and insulin levels.

The keto diet or the ketogenic diet requires you to follow a meal plan that is low in carbs and high in fat. It has some similarities with diet plans like the Atkin's diet and other low-carb meal plans. The goal of this diet is to increase the fat content in the body and reducing the carbohydrate content to push your body into the ketosis state which turns you into a fat burning machine.

BENEFITS OF KETO DIET FOR WOMEN OVER 50

The Keto diet has become so popular in recent years because of the success people have noticed. Not only have they lost weight, but scientific studies show that the Keto diet can help you improve your health in many others. As when starting any new diet or exercise routine, there may seem to be some disadvantages, so we will go over those for the Keto diet. But most people agree that the benefits outweigh the change period!

Losing Weight

For most people, this is the foremost benefit of switching to Keto! Their previous diet method may have stalled for them, or they were noticing weight creeping back on. With Keto, studies have shown that people have been able to follow this diet and relay fewer hunger pangs and suppressed appetite while losing weight at the same time! You are minimizing your carbohydrate intake, which means more occasional blood sugar spikes. Often, those fluctuations in blood sugar levels make you feel hungrier and more prone to snacking in between meals. Instead, by guiding the body towards ketosis, you are eating a more fulfilling diet of fat and protein and harnessing energy from ketone molecules instead of glucose. Studies show that low-carb diets effectively reduce visceral fat (the fat you commonly see around the abdomen increases as you become obese). This reduces your risk of obesity and improves your health in the long run.

Reduce the Risk of Type 2 Diabetes

The problem with carbohydrates is how unstable they make blood sugar levels. This can be very dangerous for people who have diabetes or are pre-diabetic because of unbalanced blood sugar levels or family history. Keto is an excellent option because of the minimal intake of carbohydrates it requires. Instead, you are harnessing most of your calories from fat or protein, which will not cause blood sugar spikes and, ultimately, less pressured the pancreas to secrete insulin. Many studies have found that diabetes patients who followed the Keto diet lost more weight and eventually reduced their fasting glucose levels. This is monumental news for patients with unstable blood sugar levels or hopes to avoid or reduce their diabetes medication intake.

Improve Cardiovascular Risk Symptoms to Lower Your Chances of Having Heart Disease

Most people assume that following Keto that is so high in fat content has to increase your risk of coronary heart disease or heart attack. But the research proves otherwise! Research shows that switching to Keto can lower your blood pressure, increase your HDL good cholesterol, and reduce your triglyceride fatty acid levels. That's because the fat you are consuming on Keto is healthy and high-quality fats, so they reverse many unhealthy symptoms of heart disease. They boost your "good" HDL cholesterol numbers and decrease your "bad" LDL cholesterol numbers. It also reduces the level of triglyceride fatty acids in the bloodstream. A top-level of these can lead to stroke, heart attack, or premature death. And what are the top levels of fatty acids linked to?

High Consumption of Carbohydrates

With the Keto diet, you are drastically cutting your intake of carbohydrates to improve fatty acid levels and improve other risk factors. A 2018 study on the Keto diet found that it can improve 22 out of 26 risk factors for cardiovascular heart disease! These factors can be critical to some people, especially those who have a history of heart disease in their family.

Increases the Body's Energy Levels

Let's briefly compare the difference between the glucose molecules synthesized from a high carbohydrate intake versus ketones produced on the Keto diet. The liver makes ketones and use fat molecules you already stored. This makes them much more energy-rich and an endless source of fuel compared to glucose, a simple sugar molecule. These ketones can give you a burst of energy physically and mentally, allowing you to have greater focus, clarity, and attention to detail.

Decreases Inflammation in the Body

Inflammation on its own is a natural response by the body's immune system, but when it becomes uncontrollable, it can lead to an array of health problems, some severe and some minor. The health concerns include acne, autoimmune conditions, arthritis, psoriasis, irritable bowel syndrome, and even acne and eczema. Often, removing sugars and carbohydrates from your diet can help patients of these diseases avoid flare-ups - and the delightful news is Keto does just that! A 2008 research study found that Keto decreased a blood marker linked to high inflammation in the body by nearly 40%. This is glorious news for people who may suffer from inflammatory disease and want to change their diet to improve.

Increases Your Mental Functioning Level

As we elaborated earlier, the energy-rich ketones can boost the body's physical and mental levels of alertness. Research has shown that Keto is a much better energy source for the brain than simple sugar glucose molecules are. With nearly 75% of your diet coming from healthy fats, the brain's neural cells and mitochondria have a better source of energy to function at the highest level. Some studies have tested patients on the Keto diet and found they had higher cognitive functioning, better memory recall, and were less susceptible to memory loss. The Keto diet can even decrease the occurrence of migraines, which can be very detrimental to patients.

Decreases Risk of Diseases like Alzheimer's, Parkinson's, and Epilepsy

They created the Keto diet in the 1920s to combat epilepsy in children. From there, research has found that Keto can improve your cognitive functioning level and protect brain cells from injury or damage. This is very good to reduce the risk of neurodegenerative disease, which begins in the brain because of neural cells mutating and functioning with damaged parts or lower than peak optimal functioning. Studies have found that the following Keto can improve the mental functioning of patients who suffer from diseases like Alzheimer's or Parkinson's. These neurodegenerative diseases sadly have no cure, but the Keto diet could improve symptoms as they progress. Researchers believe that it's because cutting out carbs from your diet, which reduces the occurrence of blood sugar spikes that the body's neural cells have to keep adjusting to.

Keto Can Regulate Hormones in Women Who Have PCOS (Polycystic Ovary Syndrome) and PMS (Pre-Menstrual Syndrome)

Women who have PCOS suffer from infertility, which can be very heartbreaking for young couples trying to start a family.

For this condition, there is no known cure, but we believe it's related to many similar diabetic symptoms like obesity and a high level of insulin. This causes the body to produce more sex hormones, which can lead to infertility. The Keto diet paved its way as a popular way to regulate insulin and hormone levels and increase a woman's chances of getting pregnant.

IMPORTANCE OF LIFESTYLE

Enhance Your Physical Activity

Taking part in physical activity may support ketone fixations during carb restriction. This effect can be improved by working in a quick paced state.

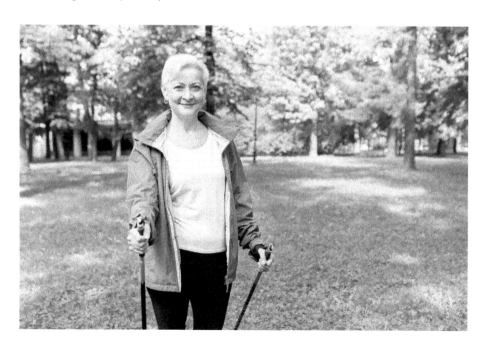

Exercising offers a plethora of benefits to all, regardless of your age! Healthy movement results in improved flexibility and more robust bones, which is quite essential for older folks. You see, as you age, your body's muscle mass starts to decrease. As we enter our fifties, adults begin to lose three to five percent of muscle mass as they enter each new decade.

However, we do realize how the thought of exercising regularly at an older age can seem like a challenge, especially if you're feeling let down with frequent aches and pains. But in many ways, the benefits of exercising outweigh the potential risks. Let's dive into why exercising is such important for seniors.

Benefits Exercising for Seniors

While you may be having thoughts about exercising, here are a couple of services that you can't ignore:

Prevents Diseases

Regular physical activity has been known to reduce the risks of diseases such as diabetes and heart disease. Mainly because exercise strengthens overall immune functioning, which is particularly beneficial for seniors who are often immunocompromised. Even if you can't hit the gym, some form of light exercise can play an integral role in disease management.

Helps Increase Social Ties and Prevents Isolation

Aging can be a daunting process, but it becomes fun when a community surrounds you. Opting for yoga or fitness classes not only makes exercising more fun, but it also helps you strengthen social ties with other older adults in your neighborhood. It can help ward off the occasional loneliness that one is likely to feel at old age. Plus, this will help you stay committed to your goals and lead a healthier lifestyle.

Improves Cognitive Function

Regular exercise can also improve fine motor skills that boost cognitive function. Several studies have shown how exercising can reduce the risk of dementia.

Tips & Tricks Exercises for Seniors

Here is a list of tips exercises that people in their fifties and beyond can enjoy:

Light Weight Training

You can start with a little weight training to retain bone

density and build muscle mass. If you're more interested in doing home exercises than joining the gym, invest in 2-pound weights, perform arm raises, and shoulder presses.

Ideally, we recommend that you join a fitness center or gym where you can meet like-minded folks. You can also get yourself a personal trainer who can guide customized workouts for you. Either way, remember to take it slow at first as you don't want to exert yourself too much.

Walking

If lifting weights isn't for you, good old-fashioned walking should also work for you. Consider taking a nice walk around your neighborhood or go to a park nearby. You'll be able to make some friends and enjoy the weather while you're at it too. In case you'd rather workout at home, strap on a pedometer, and get going around the house. You'll get more out of this workout if you move your arms and lift your knees as you take each step.

Aerobics

Joining an aerobics class can significantly help you keep your muscles healthy while maintaining mobility. It will not only improve balance but will reduce the risk of falls, thus drastically improving the overall quality of your life as you grow older.

Many studies have also indicated how aerobic exercises can protect memory and sharpen your mind and improving cognitive function among older adults. If you're not comfortable joining a class, you'll find plenty of videos online. Aerobic exercises have also been known to get the heart pumping, improving cardiovascular help.

Swimming

Do you find regular exercise too dull? Swimming is a fun, impact-free exercise that can get yours through the day. It's almost pain-free and won't trouble your aging joints. Swimming offers resistance training and will help you get back up to your feet again. Here's how it works: the water offers gentle resistance while giving you a cardiovascular workout too. It also builds muscle capacity and helps you build strength again.

Yoga

What's no to love about yoga? It's relaxing, it's healthy, and you can enjoy it with a group. Yoga does an excellent job of improving flexibility in your joints. It allows seniors to remain limber and maintain their sense of balance. If you have trouble moving about or stretching, then you can try chair yoga.

Some classic yoga poses that you might want to try out include seated forward bend, downward facing dog, and warrior.

Squats

When you're working on an exercise program, you shouldn't skip the idea of strength training. Squats happen to be an excellent way to strengthen the muscles of your lower body. Doing squats is relatively easy, and you won't need any sort of equipment except for maybe a chair to support yourself. However, if you have trouble with balance, we suggest you skip this exercise and opt for something much more straightforward.

Sit-Ups

It strengthens your core muscles, improves back pain problems, and balance. Performing simple sit-ups should do the job. You should feel the sensation in your core muscles.

WHAT FOODS CAN BE EATEN IN THE KETO DIET AND WHY

Now that we have gotten to the exciting part, it is time to learn what you can and cannot eat while following your new diet. Up until this point, you have most likely followed the food pyramid stating the importance of fruits and vegetables. While they are still going to be important for vitamins and nutrients, you are going to have to be selective. Below, you will find a complete list of foods you get to enjoy on the ketogenic diet!

Keto-Friendly Vegetables

Vegetables can be tricky when you are first starting the ketogenic diet. Some vegetables hold more carbohydrates than others. The simple rule that you need to remember is above the ground is good; below the ground is bad — got that?

Some popular above-ground vegetables you should consider for your diet (starting from the least carbs to the most carbs) include:

- Spinach
- Lettuce
- Avocado
- Asparagus

- Olives
- Cucumber
- Tomato
- Eggplant
- Cabbage
- Zucchini
- Cauliflower
- Kale
- Green Beans
- Broccoli
- Peppers
- Brussel Sprouts

And the below-ground vegetables you should avoid include:

- Carrots
- Onion
- Parsnip
- Beetroot
- Rutabaga
- Potato
- Sweet Potato

Every food that you put on your plate is comprised of three macronutrients: fat, protein, and carbohydrates. This will be an important lesson to learn before you begin your new diet, so be sure to take your time learning how to calculate them.

The golden rule is that meat and dairy are mostly made from protein and fat. Vegetables are mostly carbohydrates. Remember that while following the ketogenic diet, less than 5% of your calories need to come from carbohydrates. This is probably one of the trickiest tasks to get down when you are first getting started; there are hidden carbs everywhere! You will be amazed at how fast 20 g of carbs will go in a single day, much less a single meal!

When you are first getting started, you may want to dip your toes into the carb-cutting. As a rule, vegetables that have less than 5 net carbs can be eaten fairly freely. To make them a bit more ketogenic, I suggest putting butter on your vegetables to get a source of fat into your meal.

If you still struggle at the store, figuring out which vegetables are ketogenic, look for vegetables with leaves. Vegetables that have left are typically spinach and lettuce, both that are keto-friendly. Another rule to follow is to look for green vegetables. Generally, green vegetables like green bell peppers and green cabbage are going to be lower in carbs!

Keto-Friendly Fruits

Much like with the vegetables, some berries and fruits contain hidden carbs. As a general rule, the larger the amount of fruit, the more sugar it contains; this is why fruit is seen as nature's candy! On the ketogenic diet, that is a no go. While berries are going to be okay in moderation, the best is you leave the other fruits out for best results.

You may be thinking to yourself; I need to eat fruits for nutrients! The truth is, you can get the same nutrients from vegetables, costing you fewer carbohydrates on the ketogenic diet. While eating some berries every once in a while won't knock you out of ketosis, it is good to see how they affect you. But, if you feel like indulging in fruit as a treat, you can try some of the following:

- Raspberries
- Blackberries
- Strawberries
- Plum
- Kiwi
- Cherries
- Blueberries

- Clementine
- Cantaloupe
- Peach

Keto-Friendly Meat

On the ketogenic diet, meat is going to become a staple for you! When you are selecting your meats, try to stick with organic, grass-fed, and unprocessed. What I do want you to keep in mind is that the ketogenic diet is not meant to be high in protein, it is meant to be high in fat. People often link the ketogenic diet to a high meat diet, and that simply is not true. As you begin your diet, there is no need to have excess amounts of meat or protein. If you do have excess protein, it is going to be converted to glucose, knocking you right out of ketosis.

There are several different proteins that you will be able to enjoy while following the ketogenic diet. When it comes to beef, you will want to try your best to stick with the fattier cuts. Some of the better cuts would include ground beef, roast, veal, and steak. If poultry is more your style, look for the darker, fattier meats. Some good options for poultry selection would be wild game, turkey, duck, quail, and good old-fashioned chicken. Other options include:

- Pork Loin
- Tenderloin
- Pork Chops
- Ham
- Bacon

On your new diet, you will also be able to enjoy several different seafood dishes! At the store, you will want to look for wild-caught sources. Some of the better options include mahi-mahi, catfish, cod, halibut, trout, sardines, salmon, tuna, and mackerel. If shellfish is more your style, you get to enjoy lobster, muscles, crab, clams, and even oysters!

Keep in mind that when selecting your meats, try to avoid the cured and processed meats. These items, such as jerky, hot dogs, salami, and pepperoni, have many artificial ingredients, additives, and unnecessary sugars that will keep you from reaching ketosis. You know the better options now, stick with them!

Keto-Friendly Nuts

As you begin the ketogenic diet, there is a common misconception that you will now be able to eat as many nuts as you would like because they are high in fat. While you can enjoy a healthy serving of nuts, it is possible to go too nuts on nuts. Much like with the fruits and the vegetables, you would be surprised to learn that there are hidden carbohydrates here, too!

The lowest carb nuts you are going to find include macadamia nuts, brazil nuts, and pecans. These are fairly low in carbohydrates and can be enjoyed freely while following the ketogenic diet. These are all great options if you are looking for a healthy, ketogenic snack or something to toss in your salad.

When you are at the shop, you will want to avoid the nuts that have been treated with glazes and sugars. All of these extra add sugar and carbohydrates, which you are going to want to avoid. The higher carb nuts include cashews, pistachios, almonds, pine, and peanuts. These nuts can be enjoyed in moderation, but it would be better to avoid.

The issue with eating nuts is that it is easy to overindulge in them. While they are technically keto-friendly, they still contain a high number of calories. With that in mind, you should only be eating when you are hungry and need energy. On the ketogenic diet, you will want to avoid snacking between meals. You don't need the nuts, but they taste good! If you want to lose weight, put the nuts down, and stick to a healthier snack instead.

Keto-Friendly Snacks

On the topic of snacks, let's take a look at keto-friendly ones to have instead of a handful of nuts! Before we begin, keep in mind that if you are looking to lose weight, you will want to avoid snacking when possible. In the beginning, it may be tougher, but as you adapt to the keto diet, your meals should keep your hunger at bay for much longer.

If you are looking for something small to take the edge off your hunger pangs, look for easy whole foods, some of these basics would include eggs, cheese, cold cuts, avocados, and even olives. As long as you have these basics in your fridge, it should stop you from reaching for the high-carb foods.

If you are looking for a snack with more of a crunch, vegetable sticks are always a great option! There are plenty of dipping sauces to add fat to your meal, as well. On top of that, pork rinds are a delicious, zero-carb treat. Beef jerky is also a good option, as long as you are aware of how many carbohydrates are in a commercial package.

With the good options in mind, it's always good to take a look at the bad. When you are snacking, avoid the high-carb fruits, the coffee with creamer, and the sugar-juices. Before you started the ketogenic diet, these were probably the easy option. You'll also want to avoid the obvious candy, chips, and donuts. Just remember when you are selecting your foods, ask if it is fueling you or not.

Keto-Friendly Oils, Sauces, and Fats

On the ketogenic diet, the key to getting enough fat into your diet is going to depend on the sauces and oils you use with your cooking. When you put enough fat into your meals, this is what is going to keep you satisfied after every meal. The secret here is to be careful with the labels. You may be surprised to learn that some of your favorite condiments may have hidden sugars (looking at you, ketchup).

While you are going to have to be a bit more careful about your condiments, you can never go wrong with butter! Up until this point, you have probably been encouraged to consume a low-fat diet. Now, I want you to embrace the fat! You can put butter in absolutely anything! Put butter on your vegetables, stick it in your coffee and get creative!

Oils, on the other hand, can be a bit more complicated. You see, natural oils such as fish oil, sesame oil, almond oil, ghee, pure olive oil, and even peanut oil can be used on absolutely anything. What you want to avoid are the oils that have been created in the past sixty years or so. The oils you'll want to avoid include soy oil, corn oil, sunflower oil, and any vegetable oil. Unfortunately, these oils have been highly processed and may hinder your process.

Stick with these for your diet instead:

- Butter
- Vinaigrette
- Coconut Oil
- Mayo
- Mustard
- Guacamole
- Heavy Cream
- Thousand Island Dressing
- Salsa
- Blue Cheese Dressing
- Ranch Dip
- Pesto

When it comes to dairy, high fat is going to be your best

option. Cheese and butter are great options but keep the yogurts in moderation. When it comes to milk, you will want to avoid that as there is extra sugar in milk. If you enjoy heavy cream, this can be excellent for your cooking but should be used sparingly in your coffee.

Keto-Friendly Beverage

Remember that staying hydrated, especially when you are first starting your new diet, is going to be vital! Your safest bet is to always stick with water. Whether you like your water sparkling or flat, this is always going to be a zero-carb option. If you are struggling with a headache or the keto fly, remember that you can always throw a dash of salt in there.

WHAT FOODS TO AVOID IN THE KETO DIET AND WHY?

Because the diet is a keto, that means you need to avoid high-carbs food. Some of the food you avoid is even healthy, but it just contains too many carbs. Here is a list of typical food you should limit or avoid altogether.

Bread and Grains

No matter what form bread takes, they still pack a lot of carbs. The same applies to wholegrain as well because they are made from refined flour. So, if you want to eat bread, it is best to make keto variants at home instead. Grains such as rice, wheat, and oats pack a lot of carbs as well. So, limit or avoid that as well.

Fruits

Fruits are healthy for you. The problem is that some of those foods pack quite a lot of carbs such as banana, raisins, dates, mango, and pear. As a general rule, avoid sweet and dried fruits.

Vegetables

Vegetables are just as healthy for your body. For one, they make you feel full for longer, so they help suppress your appetite. But that also means you need to avoid or limit vegetables that are high in starch because they have more carbs than fiber. That includes corn, potato, sweet potato, and beets.

Pasta

As with any other convenient food, pasta is rich in carbs. So, spaghetti or any different types of pasta are not recommended when you are on your keto diet.

Cereal

Cereal is also a considerable offender because sugary breakfast cereals pack a lot of carbs. That also applies to "healthy cereals." Just because they use other words to describe their product does not mean that you should believe them. That also applies to oatmeal, whole-grain cereals, etc.

Beer

In reality, you can drink most alcoholic beverages in moderation without fear. Beer is an exception to this rule because it packs a lot of carbs. Carbs in beers or other liquid are considered liquid carbs, and they are even more dangerous than substantial carbs.

Sweetened Yogurt

Yogurt is very healthy because it is tasty and does not have that many carbs. The problem comes when you consume yogurt variants rich in carbs such as fruit-flavored, low-fat, sweetened, or nonfat yogurt. A single serving of sweetened yogurt contains as many carbs as a single serving of dessert.

Juice

Fruit juices are perhaps the worst beverage you can put into your system when you are on a keto diet. Another problem is that the brain does not process liquid carbs the same way as stable carbs. Substantial carbs can help suppress appetite, but liquid carbs will only put your need into overdrive.

Low-fat and fat-free salad dressings

If you have to buy salads, keep in mind that commercial sauces pack more carbs than you think, especially the fat-free and low-fat variants.

Beans and Legumes

These are also very nutritious as they are rich in fiber. However, they are also rich in carbs. You may enjoy a small amount of them when you are on your keto diet, but don't exceed your carb limit.

Sugar

We mean sugar in any form, including honey. Foods that contain lots of sugar, such as cookies, candies, and cake, are forbidden on a keto diet or any other form of diet that is designed to lose weight. When you are on a keto diet, you need to keep in mind that your diet consists of food that is rich in fiber and nutritious. So, sugar is out of the question.

Chips and Crackers

These two are some of the most popular snacks. Some people did not realize that one packet of chips contains several servings and should not be all eaten in one go. The carbs can add up very quickly if you do not watch what you eat.

Milk

Milk also contains a lot of carbs on its own. Therefore, avoid it if you can even though milk is a good source of many nutrients such as calcium, potassium, and other B vitamins.

Gluten-Free Baked Goods

Gluten-free diets are trendy nowadays, but what many people don't seem to realize is that they pack quite a lot of carbs. That includes gluten-free bread, muffins, and other baked products. In reality, they contain even more carbs than their glutinous variant.

DOES KETO DIET HAVE SIDE EFFECTS?

It would be very irresponsible of me if I only tell you all the good things about the Ketogenic Diet and ignore the side effects. The truth is that there are negative effects that could happen once you start the Ketogenic Diet – but that's actually true for all of them! All types of diet have negative effects to start with because your body has gotten used to bad habits. Once you make the shift to a more positive way of eating, the body sort of goes on a rebellious phase so it feels like everything is going wrong. For example, a person who used to eat lots of sugar in a day can have severe headaches once they start to avoid sugar. This is a withdrawal symptom and tells you that your diet is actually making positive changes to the body – albeit it takes a little bit of pain on your part.

So, what can one expect when they make that change towards a healthy Ketogenic Diet? Here are some of the things to expect and of course – how to troubleshoot these problems.

Keto Breath

One of the most common side effects of a keto diet is bad breath. Not everyone who adopts the keto diet experiences this problem, but it is common. Bad breath comes as a result of internal metabolism processes. Your liver metabolizes the massive amounts of fat you are consuming and then converts them to ketone bodies such as acetone. These ketone bodies are broken down into smaller organizations and are then circulated inside your body. As the ketone bodies circulate, it gets into your lungs through the diffusion process, and eventually, it is exerted out through your breath.

How to Overcome Keto Breath?

You can control bad keto breath by increasing water intake. You can also get rid of this problem by practicing good oral hygiene like regularly brushing your teeth. Alternatively, you can mask ketosis odor using mints and gums. It is also advisable to eat slightly more carbs and less protein if you have this problem.

Keto Flu

You may experience symptoms resembling those of flu, especially during your first days on a keto diet. Such symptoms include aches, fatigue, cramping, skin rash, and diarrhea. The side effects are caused by dehydration as a result of your body losing a lot of water and electrolytes.

When your body uses fat to fuel its functions instead of using protein, you tend to lose more water and electrolytes through urination. The loss of water and electrolytes is accelerated further by the low insulin levels and muscle glycogen that accompanies the keto diet.

Besides, most keto diets consist of food with little water and potassium levels, further accelerating the loss of body water and electrolytes.

How to Overcome Keto Flu?

You can handle keto flu by drinking much water. You can also eat lots of soup. If you get enough rest, you will give your body enough energy to fight the flu on its own.

You need to lower the effects of keto flu by getting enough sleep. You can also drink much water to minimize the impact of keto flu. There are also some supplements found in natural sources like organic coffee or matcha tea that could help you overcome the flu. Make a point to get enough salts and electrolytes, too.

Fatigue

You may experience extreme feelings of tiredness once you adopt a keto diet. Fatigue is caused by a lack of glucose reaching your brain. Although this side effect will last for a few days, it could still cause much discomfort and worry on your part.

How to Overcome Keto Fatigue?

Drink much water and get enough rest. You can also avoid engaging in strenuous exercises. You can also eat healthy carbs to give you the extra energy your body needs.

GI Side Effects

Keto diet can also harm your digestive system over the long term. Keto diet has been thought to cause some stomach problems such as constipation high cholesterol levels, diarrhea, kidneys stones, and vomiting.

You may also experience abnormal stomach gas due to the sugar alcohols found in some keto diets, for example, the sugars found in some processed foods. The higher the amount of food you eat, the higher the impact of the side effects on you.

How to Control GI Problems When You Are on a Keto Diet?

Drink lots of water and eat high fiber foods such as fruits and vegetables to encourage the growth of beneficial bacteria in your GI system. Make it a habit of exercising regularly.

Weakened Immune System

Keto diets can also weaken the immune systems of some people. Studies suggest that keto foods could cause a condition called dysbiosis. Dysbiosis occurs when the balance of helpful and harmful bacteria is altered in your GI tract. The disruption is caused by the consumption of highly saturated fats and low fiber levels in your digestive system.

When you ingest diets with little prebiotic fiber, the number of beneficial bacteria decreases substantially in your digestive system. Your GI tract is the backbone of your immune system, and any compromise to it could have a negative impact on the immune functions leading to exposure to chronic diseases.

How to Avoid Weakened Immune System When on a Keto Diet?

Incorporate workouts to your keto diet. You can also eat high fiber food, such as fruits and vegetables. Also, ensure you drink lots of water.

Vitamin and Other Mineral Deficiencies

If you are on the keto diet, you may not receive enough vitamins and minerals needed for your body to function normally. Plant-based minerals such as calcium and vitamin D may not be present in your keto diet in the quantities required by your body. If these minerals decrease in your body for long periods, you may stand a high risk of getting lifestyle diseases such as heart failure.

Heart failure comes as a result of the hardening of your heart muscles because of the lack of enough selenium. Selenium is an essential immune-boosting antioxidant usually occurring in plant-based food. Lack of this critical antioxidant causes the hardening of your heart muscles leading to heart failure.

How to Treat the Deficiencies When You Are on a Keto Diet?

Eat lots of fruits and vegetables to get vitamins. You can also use beneficial supplements to treat any deficiencies, which comes with the keto diet.

Increased Risk of Chronic Disease

The Keto diet requires you to put a limit on the number of carbohydrates and protein you consume. When you eat much fat to get enough calories needed by your body, you will be limiting fiber-rich foods such as vegetables, fruits, or legumes. These foods are some of the best sources of immune-boosting nutrients needs by your body to stay healthy. Therefore, when you limit these nutrients in your body, you increase your risk of getting chronic diseases such as diabetes, cancer, high blood pressure.

Studies show that diets that are high in fruits and vegetables can significantly reduce chronic diseases. The more you consume them, the better you are health-wise. When you restrict their consumption, you tend to decrease their beneficial impacts.

How to Reduce the Risk of Chronic Diseases When on Keto Diets?

We'll say it again: drink lots of water. Eat lots of fruits and vegetables. You can also incorporate exercise into your keto diet to get the best results.

Chronic Inflammation

Studies show that when you consume high fats needed for Ketosis, your cholesterol and lipoprotein structure could be significantly altered and will result in inflammation over a while. Inflammation occurs when the cells of your body use much energy to accomplish their normal functioning. Chronic inflammation is also one of the causes of heart diseases.

How to Minimize Chronic Inflammation When on Keto Diets?

You can control the problem of inflammation by eating solid fats and oils. Ensure you also include high fiber foods in your daily intake, like fruits and vegetables.

The Challenge of Weight Cycling

When you restrict your eating diets for an extended period, you may end up gaining too much weight when not dieting, which you then go ahead and lose when on a diet. This process of alternating between weight gain and weight loss is what is referred to as weight cycling. Weight cycling can increase the risk of getting chronic diseases.

How to Control Weight Cycling?

You can control weight cycling by shortening the intervals between dieting and the days you are on free diets. You should gradually increase the amount of food you consume during your free diet days so that your body can have enough time to adjust to the changes in your program.

BREAKFAST

RECIPES

Yogurt Waffles

Prep Time:	Cooking Time:	Servings:
15 min	25 min	4

Ingredients:

- ½ cup golden flax seeds meal
- ½ cup plus 3 tablespoons almond flour
- 1½ tbsp. granulated erythritol
- 1 tbsp. unsweetened vanilla whey protein powder
- ½ tsp. organic powder
- ¼ tsp. xanthan gum
- Salt, to taste
- 1 large organic egg, white and yolk separated
- 1 organic whole egg
- 2 tbsp. unsweetened almond milk
- 1½ tbsp. unsalted butter
- 3 oz. plain Greek yogurt
- ¼ tsp. baking soda.

Directions:

Preheat the waffle iron and then grease it.

In a large bowl, add the flour, erythritol, protein powder, baking soda, baking powder, xanthan gum, salt, and mix until well combined.

In a second small bowl, add the egg white and beat until stiff peaks form.

In a third bowl, add 2 egg yolks, whole egg, almond milk, butter, yogurt and beat until well combined.

Place egg mixture into the bowl of flour mixture and mix until well combined.

Gently, fold in the beaten egg whites.

Place ¼ cup of the mixture into preheated waffle iron and cook for about 4–5 minutes or until golden-brown.

Repeat with the remaining mixture.

Serve warm.

Nutrition:

Calories: 250 kcal | Carbs: 3.2 g | Total Carbs: 8.8 g | Fiber: 5.6 g | Sugar: 1.3 g | Protein 8.4 g

Broccoli Muffins

Prep Time:	Cooking Time:	Servings:
15 min	20 min	5

Ingredients:

- 2 tbsp. unsalted butter
- 6 large organic eggs
- ½ cup heavy whipping cream
- ½ cup Parmesan cheese, grated
- Salt and ground black pepper, to taste
- 1¼ cup broccoli, chopped
- 2 tbsp. fresh parsley, chopped

- ½ cup Swiss cheese, grated.

Directions:

Preheat your oven to 350°F.

Grease a 12-cup muffin tin.

In a bowl, add the eggs, cream, Parmesan cheese, salt, black pepper and beat until well combined.

Divide the broccoli and parsley in the bottom of each prepared muffin cup evenly.

Top with the egg mixture, followed by the Swiss cheese.

Bake for about 20 minutes, rotating the pan once halfway through.

Remove from the oven and place onto a wire rack for about 5 minutes before serving.

Carefully, invert the muffins onto a serving platter and serve warm.

Nutrition:

Calories: 231 kcal | Total Carbs: 2.5 g | Fiber: 0.5 g | Sugar: 0.9 g | Protein: 13.5 g.

Spinach Artichoke Breakfast Bake

Prep Time:	Cooking Time:	Servings:
15 min	20 min	7

Ingredients:

- ¼ cup milk, fat-free
- ¼ tsp. ground pepper
- ⅓ cup red pepper, diced
- ½ cup feta cheese crumbles
- ½ cup scallions, finely sliced
- ¾ cup canned artichokes, chopped, drained, & patted dry
- 1¼ tsp. kosher salt
- 1 clove garlic, minced
- 1 tbsp. dill, chopped
- 10 oz. spinach, frozen, chopped & drained
- 2 tbsp. parmesan cheese, grated
- 4 large egg whites
- 8 large eggs.

Directions:

Preheat the oven to 375°F and grease a large baking dish with nonstick spray or preferred fat source.

In a small bowl, combine the spinach, artichoke, scallions,

garlic, red pepper, and fill.

Combine completely and then pour into the baking dish, spreading into an even layer.

In a mixing bowl, combine eggs, egg whites, salt, pepper, parmesan, and milk.

Whisk until completely combined, then add feta and mix once more.

Pour the egg mixture evenly over the vegetables in the baking dish.

Bake for about 35 minutes, until a butter knife inserted in the center comes out clean.

Allow to cool for about 10 minutes before cutting into eight equal pieces.

Serve warm!

Nutrition:

Calories: 574 kcal | Carbs: 2 g | Fiber: 0.7 g | Sugar: 0.1 g | Protein: 47 g | Fat: 54 g | Sodium: 254 mg.

Granola Bars

Prep Time:	Cooking Time:	Servings:
15 min	20 min	6

Ingredients:

- 2 cups almonds, chopped
- ½ cup pumpkin seeds, raw
- ⅓ cup coconut flakes, unsweetened
- 2 tbsp. hemp seeds
- ¼ cup clear Sukrin Fiber Syrup
- ¼ cup almond butter
- ¼ cup erythritol, powdered, or equal measure of preferred sweetener
- 2 tsp. vanilla extract
- ½ tsp. sea salt.

Directions:

Line a small, square baking dish with parchment paper.

In a mixing bowl, combine almonds, pumpkin seeds, coconut flakes, and hemp seeds. Stir until evenly mixed.

Over medium heat combine the syrup, almond butter, sweetener, salt, and stir until it's smooth and easy to pull the spoon through.

Remove the pan from the heat and stir the vanilla extract into the mixture.

Pour the syrup over the seeds and stir completely.

Pour the mixture into the baking dish and press evenly into one layer and press until the top is even.

Let cool completely and slice into 12 bars.

Nutrition:

Calories: 254 kcal | Carbs: 2 g | Sugar: 0.1 g | Fiber: 0.7 g | Protein: 42.5 g | Fat: 47 g | Sodium: 145

Pumpkin Bread

Prep Time:	Cooking Time:	Servings:
15 min	1 h	5

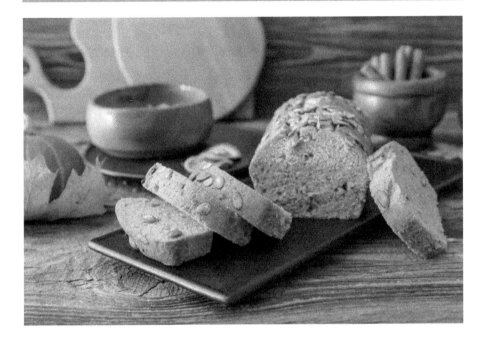

Ingredients:

- 1⅔ cup almond flour
- 1½ tsp. organic baking powder
- ½ tsp. pumpkin pie spice
- ½ tsp. ground cinnamon
- ½ tsp. ground cloves
- ½ tsp. salt
- 8 oz. cream cheese, softened

- 6 organic eggs, divided
- 1 tbsp. coconut flour
- 1 cup powdered erythritol, divided
- 1 tsp. stevia powder, divided
- 1 tsp. organic lemon extract
- 1 cup homemade pumpkin puree
- ½ cup coconut oil, melted

Directions:

Preheat your oven to 325ºF.

Lightly, grease 2 bread loaf pans.

In a bowl, place almond flour, baking powder, spices, salt and mix until well combined.

In a second bowl, add the cream cheese, 1 egg, coconut flour, ¼ cup of erythritol, ¼ teaspoon of the stevia and with a wire whisk, beat until smooth.

In a third bowl, add the pumpkin puree, oil, 5 eggs, ¾ cup of the erythritol, ¾ teaspoon of the stevia, and with a wire whisk, beat until well combined.

Add the pumpkin mixture into the bowl of the flour mixture and mix until just combined.

Place about ¼ of the pumpkin mixture into each loaf pan

evenly.

Top each pan with the cream cheese mixture evenly, followed by the remaining pumpkin mixture.

Bake for about 50–60 minutes or until a toothpick inserted in the center comes out clean.

Remove the bread pans from oven and place onto a wire rack and let it be for 10 minutes.

With a sharp knife, cut each bread loaf in the desired-sized slices and serve.

Nutrition:

Calories: 216 kcal | Total Carbs: 4.5 g | Fiber: 2 g | Sugar: 1.1 g | Protein: 3.4 g.

LUNCH

RECIPES

Lettuce Salad

Prep Time:	Cooking Time:	Servings:
10 min	0 min	1

Ingredients:

- 1 cup Romaine lettuce, roughly chopped
- 3 oz. seitan, chopped
- 1 tbsp. avocado oil
- 1 tsp. sunflower seeds
- 1 tsp. lemon juice
- 1 egg, boiled, peeled
- 2 oz. Cheddar cheese, shredded.

Directions:

Place lettuce in the salad bowl. Add chopped seitan and shredded cheese. Then chop the egg roughly and add in the salad bowl too. Mix up together lemon juice with the avocado oil. Sprinkle the salad with the oil mixture and sunflower seeds. Don't stir the salad before serving.

Nutrition:

Calories: 20 kcal | Fat: 0.2 g | Carbs: 4.2 g | Protein: 1.2 g.

Pita Pizza

Prep Time:	Cooking Time:	Servings:
15 min	10 min	2

Ingredients:

- ½ cup marinara sauce
- 1 low-carb pita
- 2 oz. cheddar cheese
- 14 slices pepperoni
- 1 oz. roasted red peppers.

Directions:

Program the oven temperature setting to 450°F.

Slice the pita in half and place onto a foil-lined baking tray.

Rub with a bit of oil and toast for one to two minutes.

Pour the sauce over the bread.

Sprinkle using the cheese and other toppings.

Bake until the cheese melts (5 minutes). Cool thoroughly.

Nutrition:

Calories: 250 kcal | Carbs: 4 g | Protein: 13 g | Fats: 19 g.

Creamy Zoodles

Prep Time:	Cooking Time:	Servings:
15 min	10 min	4

Ingredients:

- 1¼ cups heavy whipping cream
- ¼ cup mayonnaise
- Salt and ground black pepper, as required
- 30 oz. zucchini, spiralized with blade C
- 3 oz. Parmesan cheese, grated
- 2 tbsp. fresh mint leaves
- 2 tbsp. butter, melted.

Directions:

The heavy cream must be added to a pan then bring to a boil.

Lower the heat to low and cook until reduced in half.

Put in the pepper, mayo, and salt; cook until mixture is warm enough.

Add the zucchini noodles and gently stir to combine.

Stir in the Parmesan cheese.

Divide the zucchini noodles onto four serving plates and immediately drizzle with the melted butter.

Serve immediately.

Nutrition:

Calories: 241 kcal| Fat: 11.4 g | Fiber: 7.5 g | Carbs: 3.1 g | Protein: 5.1 g.

Cheesy Bacon Squash Spaghetti

Prep Time:	Cooking Time:	Servings:
30 min	50 min	4

Ingredients:

- 2 pounds spaghetti squash
- 2 pounds bacon
- ½ cup of butter
- 2 cups of shredded parmesan cheese
- Salt
- Black pepper.

Directions:

Let the oven preheat to 375ºF.

Trim or remove each stem of spaghetti squash, slice into rings no more than an inch wide, and take out the seeds.

Lay the sliced rings down on the baking sheet, bake for 40-45 minutes.

It is ready when the strands separate easily when a fork is used to scrape it. Let it cool.

Cook sliced up bacon until crispy. Take out and let it cool.

Take off the shell on each ring, separate each strand with a fork, and put them in a bowl.

Heat the strands in a microwave to get them warm, then put in butter and stir around till the butter melts.

Pour in parmesan cheese and bacon crumbles and add salt and pepper to your taste. Enjoy.

Nutrition:

Calories: 398 kcal | Fat: 12.5 g | Fiber: 9.4 g | Carbs: 4.1 g | Protein: 5.1 g.

Mushroom & Cauliflower Risotto

Prep Time:	Cooking Time:	Servings:
5 min	10 min	4

Ingredients:

- 1 grated head of cauliflower
- 1 cup vegetable stock
- 9 oz. chopped mushrooms
- 2 tbsp. butter
- 1 cup coconut cream.

Directions:

Pour the stock in a saucepan. Boil and set aside.

Prepare a skillet with butter and sauté the mushrooms until golden.

Grate and stir in the cauliflower and stock.

Simmer and add the cream, cooking until the cauliflower is al dente.

Serve.

Nutrition:

Calories: 186 kcal | Carbs: 4 g | Protein: 1 g | Fats: 17 g.

Salmon Pasta

Prep Time:	Cooking Time:	Servings:
15 min	1 h 30 min	2

Ingredients:

- 2 tbsp. Coconut oil
- 2 zucchinis
- 8 oz. Smoked salmon
- ¼ cup Keto-friendly mayo

Directions:

Make noodle-like strands from the zucchini.

Warm-up, the oil, put the salmon and sauté within 2 to 3 minutes.

Stir in the noodles and sauté for 1 to 2 more minutes.

Stir in the mayo and serve.

Nutrition:

Calories: 470 kcal | Carbs: 3 g | Protein: 21 g | Fats: 42 g.

Taco Casserole

Prep Time:	Cooking Time:	Servings:
10 min	20 min	8

Ingredients:

- 1½ to 2 lb. ground turkey or beef
- 2 tbsp. taco seasoning
- 8 oz. shredded cheddar cheese
- 1 cup salsa
- 16 oz. cottage cheese.

Directions:

Heat the oven to reach 400 °F.

Combine the taco seasoning and ground meat in a casserole dish.

Bake it for 20 minutes.

Combine the salsa and both kinds of cheese. Set aside for now.

Carefully transfer the casserole dish from the oven.

Drain away the cooking juices from the meat.

Break the meat into small pieces and mash with a masher or fork.

Sprinkle with cheese.

Bake in the oven for 15 to 20 more minutes until the top is browned.

Nutrition:

Calories: 367 kcal | Carbs: 6 g | Protein: 45 g | Fats: 18 g.

Beef Wellington

Prep Time:	Cooking Time:	Servings:
20 min	40 min	4

Ingredients:

- 2 (4-ounce) grass-fed beef tenderloin steaks, halved
- Salt and ground black pepper, as required
- 1 tbsp. butter
- 1 cup mozzarella cheese, shredded
- ½ cup almond flour
- 4 tbsp. liver pate.

Directions:

Preheat your oven to 400°F.

Grease a baking sheet.

Season the steaks with pepper and salt.

Sear the beef steaks for about 2–3 minutes per side.

In a microwave-safe bowl, add the mozzarella cheese and microwave for about 1 minute.

Remove from the microwave and stir in the almond flour until a dough forms.

Place the dough between 2 parchment paper pieces and, with a rolling pin, roll to flatten it.

Remove the upper parchment paper piece.

Divide the rolled dough into four pieces.

Place one tablespoon of pate onto each dough piece and top with one steak piece.

Cover each steak piece with dough completely.

Arrange the covered steak pieces onto the prepared baking sheet in a single layer.

Baking time: 20-30 minutes.

Serve warm.

Nutrition:

Calories: 412 kcal| Fat: 15.6g | Carbs: 4.9 g | Fiber: 9.1g | Protein: 18.5g.

Keto Croque Monsieur

Prep Time:	Cooking Time:	Servings:
5 min	7 min	2

Ingredients:

- 2 eggs
- ¾ oz. of grated cheese
- ¾ oz. of ham 1 large slice
- 3 tbsp. of cream
- 3 tbsp. of mascarpone
- 1 oz. of butter
- Pepper and salt
- Basil leaves, optional, to garnish.

Directions:

Carefully crack eggs in a neat bowl, add some salt and pepper.

Add the cream, mascarpone, grated cheese, and stir together.

Melt the butter over medium heat. The butter must not turn brown.

Once the butter has melted, set the heat to low.

Add half of the omelette mixture to the frying pan and then immediately place the slice of ham on it.

Now pour the rest of the omelette mixture over the ham and then immediately put a lid on it.

Allow it to fry for 2-3 minutes over low heat until the top is slightly firmer.

Slide the omelette onto the lid to turn the omelette.

Then put the omelette back in the frying pan to fry for another 1-2 minutes on the other side (still on low heat), then put the lid back on the pan.

Don't let the omelette cook for too long!

It does not matter if it is still liquid.

Garnish with a few basil leaves if necessary.

Nutrition:

Calories: 479 kcal | Protein: 16 g | Fats: 45 g | Carbs: 4 g.

Sesame Pork with Green Beans

Prep Time:	Cooking Time:	Servings:
5 min	10 min	2

Ingredients:

- 2 boneless pork chops
- Pink Himalayan salt
- Freshly ground black pepper
- 2 tbsp. toasted sesame oil, divided
- 2 tbsp. soy sauce
- 1 tsp. Sriracha sauce
- 1 cup fresh green beans.

Directions:

On a cutting board, pat the pork chops dry with a paper towel. Slice the chops into strips and season with pink Himalayan salt and pepper.

In a large skillet over medium heat, heat one tablespoon of sesame oil.

Add the pork strips and cook them for 7 minutes, stirring occasionally.

In a small bowl, mix the remaining one tablespoon of

sesame oil, the soy sauce, and the Sriracha sauce. Pour into the skillet with the pork.

Add the green beans to the skillet, reduce the heat to medium-low, and simmer for 3 to 5 minutes.

Divide the pork, green beans, and sauce between two wide, shallow bowls and serve.

Nutrition:

Calories: 387 kcal | Fat: 15.1 g | Carbs: 4.1 g | Fiber: 10 g | Protein: 18.1 g

Pan-Seared Cod with Tomato Hollandaise

Prep Time:	Cooking Time:	Servings:
10 min	10 min	4

Ingredients:

- Pan-Seared Cod
- 1 pound (4-fillets) wild Alaskan Cod
- 1 tbsp. salted butter
- 1 tbsp. olive oil
- Tomato Hollandaise
- 3 large egg yolks
- 3 tbsp. warm water
- 8 oz. salted butter, melted
- ¼ tsp. salt
- ¼ tsp. black pepper
- 2 tbsp. tomato paste
- 2 tbsp. fresh lemon juice.

Directions:

Season both sides of the code fillet without salt, the salt will be added in the last.

Heat a skillet over medium heat and coat with olive oil and butter.

When the butter heats up, place the cod fillet in the skillet and sear on both sides for 2-3 minutes. Baste the fish fillet with the oil and butter mixture.

You will know that the cod cooked when it easily flakes when poked with a fork.

Melt the butter in the microwave.

In a double boil, beat egg yolks with warm water until thick and creamy and start forming soft peaks. Remove the double boil from the heat, gradually adding the melted butter and stirring.

Season.

Mix in the tomato paste. Stir to combine. Pour in the water and lemon juice to lighten the sauce texture.

Nutrition:

Calories: 356 | Fat: 16.1 g | Carbs: 3.1 g | Fiber: 12.3 g | Protein: 18.4 g.

Creamy Scallops

Prep Time:	Cooking Time:	Servings:
10 min	10 min	4

Ingredients:

- 1 lb. scallops, rinse and pat dry
- 1 tsp. fresh parsley, chopped
- ⅛ tsp. cayenne pepper
- 2 tbsp. white wine
- ¼ cup water
- 3 tbsp. heavy cream
- 1 tsp. garlic, minced
- 1 tbsp. butter, melted
- 1 tbsp. olive oil
- Pepper
- Salt.

Direction:

Season scallops with pepper and salt.

Heat butter and oil in a pan over medium heat.

Add scallops and sear until browned from both sides. Transfer scallops on a plate.

Add garlic in the same pan and sauté for 30 seconds.

Add water, heavy cream, wine, cayenne pepper, and salt. Stir well and cook until sauce thickens.

Return scallops to pan and stir well.

Garnish with parsley and serve.

Nutrition:

Calories: 202 kcal | Fat: 11.4 g | Cholesterol: 60 mg | Carbs: 3.5 g | Sugar: 0.1 g | Protein: 19.4 g.

Easy Baked Shrimp Scampi

Prep Time:	Cooking Time:	Servings:
10 min	10 min	4

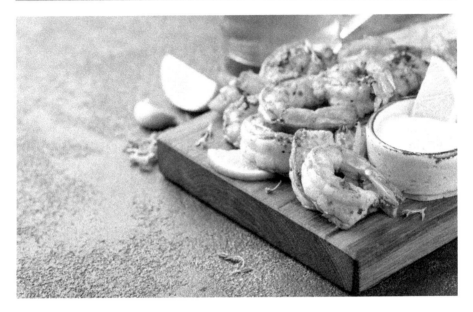

Ingredients:

- 2 lb. shrimp, peeled
- ¾ cup olive oil
- 2 tsp. dried oregano
- 1 tbsp. garlic, minced
- ½ cup fresh lemon juice
- ¼ cup butter, sliced
- Pepper
- Salt.

Directions:

Preheat the oven to 350°F.

Add shrimp in a baking dish.

In a bowl, whisk together lemon juice, oregano, garlic, oil, pepper, salt, and pour over shrimp.

Add butter on top of shrimp.

Bake in preheated oven for 10 minutes or until shrimp is cooked.

Serve and enjoy.

Nutrition:

Calories: 708 kcal | Fat: 53.5 g | Cholesterol: 508 mg | Carbs: 5.3 g | Sugar: 0.7 g | Protein: 52.2 g.

Signature Italian Pork Dish

Prep Time:	Cooking Time:	Servings:
15 min	15 min	6

Ingredients:

- 2 lb. pork tenderloins, cut into 1½-inch pieces
- ¼ cup almond flour
- 1 tsp. garlic salt
- Freshly ground black pepper, to taste
- 2 tbsp. butter
- ½ cup homemade chicken broth
- ⅓ cup balsamic vinegar
- 1 tbsp. capers
- 2 tsp. fresh lemon zest, grated finely.

Direction:

In a large bowl, add the pork pieces, flour, garlic salt, black pepper, and toss to coat well.

Remove pork pieces from bowl and shake off excess flour mixture.

In a large skillet, melt the butter over medium-high heat and cook the pork pieces for about 2-3 minutes per side.

Add broth and vinegar and bring to a gentle boil.

Reduce the heat to medium and simmer for about 3-4 minutes.

With a slotted spoon, transfer the pork pieces onto a plate.

In the same skillet, add the capers, lemon zest, and simmer for about 3-5 minutes or until the desired thickness of sauce.

Pour sauce over pork pieces and serve.

Nutrition:

Calories: 373 kcal | Carbs: 1.8 g | Fiber: 0.7 g | Sugar: 0.4 g | Protein: 46.7 g | Fat: 18.6 g | Sodium: 231 mg.

Broccoli and Chicken Casserole

Prep Time:	Cooking Time:	Servings:
15 min	35 min	6

Ingredients:

- 2 tbsp. butter
- ¼ cup cooked bacon, crumbled
- 2½ cups cheddar cheese, shredded and divided
- 4 oz. cream cheese, softened
- ¼ cup heavy whipping cream
- ½ pack ranch seasoning mix
- ⅔ cup homemade chicken broth
- 1½ cups small broccoli florets
- 2 cups cooked grass-fed chicken breast, shredded.

Directions:

Preheat your oven to 350°F.

Arrange a rack in the upper portion of the oven.

For the chicken mixture: In a large wok, melt the butter over low heat.

Add the bacon, 1/2 cup of cheddar cheese, cream cheese, heavy whipping cream, ranch seasoning, and broth, and with a wire whisk, beat until well combined.

Cook for about 5 minutes, stirring frequently.

Meanwhile, in a microwave-safe dish, place the broccoli and microwave until desired tenderness is achieved.

In the wok, add the chicken and broccoli and mix until well combined.

Remove from the heat and transfer the mixture into a casserole dish.

Top the chicken mixture with the remaining cheddar cheese.

Bake for about 25 minutes.

Now, set the oven to broiler.

Broil the chicken mixture for about 2–3 minutes or until cheese is bubbly.

Serve hot.

Nutrition:

Calories: 431 | Fat: 10.5g | Fiber: 9.1g | Carbs:4.9 g | Protein: 14.1g.

Keto Wraps with Cream Cheese and Salmon

Prep Time:	Cooking Time:	Servings:
5 min	10 min	2

Ingredients:

- 3 oz. of cream cheese
- 1 tbsp. of dill or other fresh herbs
- 1 oz. of smoked salmon
- 1 egg
- ½ oz. of butter

- Pinch of cayenne pepper
- Pepper and salt.

Directions:

Beat the egg well in a bowl. With 1 egg, you can make two thin wraps in a small frying pan.

Melt the butter over medium heat in a small frying pan.

Once the butter has melted, add half of the beaten egg to the pan.

Move the pan back and forth so that the entire bottom is covered with a very thin layer of egg. Turn down the heat!

Carefully loosen the egg on the edges with a silicone spatula and turn the wafer-thin omelets as soon as the egg is no longer dripping (about 45 seconds to 1 minute).

You can do this by sliding it onto a lid or plate and then sliding it back into the pan.

Let the other side be cooked for about 30 seconds and then remove from the pan.

The omelets must be nice and light yellow.

Repeat for the rest of the beaten egg.

Once the omelets are ready, let them cool on a cutting board or plate and make the filling.

Cut the dill into small pieces and put in a bowl

Add the cream cheese, the salmon cut into small pieces, and mix together. Add a tiny bit of cayenne pepper and mix well. Taste immediately and then season with salt and pepper.

Spread a layer on the wrap and roll it up. Cut the wrap in half and keep in the fridge until you are ready to eat it.

Nutrition:

Calories: 237 kcal | Carbs: 14.7 g | Protein: 15 g | Fat: 5 g.

DINNER RECIPES

Korma Curry

Prep Time:	Cooking Time:	Servings:
10 min	25 min	6

Ingredients:

- 3-pound chicken breast, skinless, boneless
- 1 tsp. garam masala
- 1 tsp. curry powder
- 1 tbsp. apple cider vinegar
- ½ coconut cream
- 1 cup organic almond milk
- 1 tsp. ground coriander
- ¾ tsp. ground cardamom
- ½ tsp. ginger powder
- ¼ tsp. cayenne pepper
- ¾ tsp. ground cinnamon
- 1 tomato, diced
- 1 tsp. avocado oil
- ½ cup of water.

Directions:

Chop the chicken breast and put it in the saucepan.

Add avocado oil and start to cook it over medium heat.

Sprinkle the chicken with garam masala, curry powder, apple cider vinegar, ground coriander, cardamom, ginger powder, cayenne pepper, ground cinnamon, and diced tomato. Mix up the ingredients carefully.

Cook them for 10 minutes.

Add water, coconut cream, and almond milk. Sauté the meat for 10 minutes more.

Nutrition:

Calories: 440 kcal | Fat: 32 g | Fiber: 4 g | Carbs: 28 g | Protein: 8 g.

Stuffed Portobello Mushrooms

Prep Time:	Cooking Time:	Servings:
10 min	10 min	4

Ingredients:

- 2 portobello mushrooms
- 1 cup spinach, chopped, steamed
- 2 oz. artichoke hearts, drained, chopped
- 1 tbsp. coconut cream
- 1 tbsp. cream cheese
- 1 tsp. minced garlic
- 1 tbsp. fresh cilantro, chopped
- 3 oz. Cheddar cheese, grated
- ½ tsp. ground black pepper
- 2 tbsp. olive oil
- ½ tsp. salt.

Directions:

Sprinkle mushrooms with olive oil and place in the tray.

Transfer the tray to the preheated to 360°F oven and broil them for 5 minutes.

Meanwhile, blend artichoke hearts, coconut cream, cream

cheese, minced garlic, and chopped cilantro.

Add grated cheese to the mixture and sprinkle with ground black pepper and salt.

Fill the broiled mushrooms with the cheese mixture and cook them for 5 minutes more. Serve the mushrooms only hot.

Nutrition:

Calories: 135.2 kcal | Total Fat: 5.5 g | Cholesterol: 16.4 mg | Sodium: 698.1 mg | Potassium: 275.3 mg | Carbs: 8.4 g | Protein: 14.8 g.

Italian Style Halibut Packets

Prep Time:	Cooking Time:	Servings:
10 min	20 min	4

Ingredients:

- 2 cups cauliflower florets
- 1 cup roasted red pepper strips
- ½ cup sliced sun-dried tomatoes
- 4 (4-ounce) halibut fillets
- ¼ cup chopped fresh basil
- 1 lemon juice
- ¼ cup good-quality olive oil
- Sea salt, for seasoning
- Freshly ground black pepper, for seasoning.

Directions:

Preheat the oven. Set the oven temperature to 400°F.

Make the packets.

Divide the cauliflower, red pepper strips, and sun-dried tomato between the four pieces of foil, placing the vegetables in the middle of each piece.

Top each pile with one halibut fillet and top each fillet with equal amounts of the basil, lemon juice, and olive oil.

Fold and crimp the foil to form sealed packets of fish and vegetables and place them on the baking sheet.

Bake. Bake the packets for about 20 minutes, until the fish flakes with a fork.

Be careful of the steam when you open the packet!

Serve. Transfer the vegetables and halibut to four plates, season with salt and pepper, and serve immediately.

Nutrition:

Calories: 313 kcal| Fat: 14.1 g | Carbs: 3.2 g | Fiber: 10.4 g | Protein: 15.4 g.

Pesto Flavored Steak

Prep Time:	Cooking Time:	Servings:
15 min	17 min	4

Ingredients:

- ¼ cup fresh oregano, chopped
- 1½ tbsp. garlic, minced
- 1 tbsp. fresh lemon peel, grated
- ½ tsp. red pepper flakes, crushed
- Salt and freshly ground black pepper, to taste
- 1 lb. (1-inch thick) grass-fed boneless beef top sirloin steak
- 1 cup pesto
- ¼ cup feta cheese, crumbled.

Direction:

Preheat the gas grill to medium heat. Lightly, grease the grill grate.

In a bowl, add the oregano, garlic, lemon peel, red pepper flakes, salt, black pepper, and mix well.

Rub the garlic mixture onto the steak evenly.

Place the steak onto the grill and cook, covered for about 12-

17 minutes, flipping occasionally.

Remove from the grill and place the steak onto a cutting board for about 5 minutes.

With a sharp knife, cut the steak into desired sized slices.

Divide the steak slices and pesto onto serving plates and serve with the topping of the feta cheese.

Nutrition:

Calories: 226 kcal | Carbs: 6.8 g | Sugar: 0.7 g | Fiber: 2.2 g | Protein: 40.5 g | Fat: 7.6 g | Sodium: 579 mg.

Flawless Grilled Steak

Prep Time:	Cooking Time:	Servings:
21 min	10 min	5

Ingredients:

- ½ tsp. dried thyme, crushed
- ½ tsp. dried oregano, crushed
- 1 tsp. red chili powder
- ½ tsp. ground cumin
- ¼ tsp. garlic powder
- Salt, to taste
- Freshly ground black pepper, to taste

- 1½ lb. grass-fed flank steak, trimmed
- ¼ cup Monterrey Jack cheese, crumbled.

Direction:

In a large bowl, add the dried herbs and spices and mix well.

Add the steaks and rub with mixture generously.

Set aside for about 15-20 minutes.

Preheat the grill to medium heat. Grease the grill grate.

Place the steak onto the grill over medium coals and cook for about 17-21 minutes, flipping once halfway through.

Remove the steak from the grill and place onto a cutting board for about 10 minutes before slicing.

With a sharp knife, cut the steak into desired sized slices.

Top with the cheese and serve.

Nutrition:

Calories: 271 kcal | Carbs: 0.7 g | Sugar: 0.1 g | Fiber: 0.3 g | Protein: 38.3 g | Fat: 11.8 g | Sodium: 119 mg.

Kalua Pork with Cabbage

Prep Time:	Cooking Time:	Servings:
10 min	8 h	4

Ingredients:

- 1-pound boneless pork butt roast
- Pink Himalayan salt
- Freshly ground black pepper
- 1 tbsp. smoked paprika or Liquid Smoke
- ½ cup of water
- ½ head cabbage, chopped.

Directions:

With the crock insert in place, preheat the slow cooker to low.

Generously season the pork roast with pink Himalayan salt, pepper, and smoked paprika.

Place the pork roast in the slow-cooker insert, and add the water.

Cover and cook on low for 7 hours.

Transfer the cooked pork roast to a plate. Put the chopped cabbage in the bottom of the slow cooker, and put the pork roast back in on the cabbage.

Cover and cook the cabbage and pork roast for 1 hour.

Remove the pork roast from the slow cooker and place it on a baking sheet. Use two forks to shred the pork.

Serve the shredded pork hot with the cooked cabbage.

Reserve the liquid from the slow cooker to remoisten the pork and cabbage when reheating leftovers.

Nutrition:

Calories: 451 kcal | Fat: 19.3 g | Carbs: 2.1 g | Fiber: 11.2 g | Protein: 14.3 g.

Coffee BBQ Pork Belly

Prep Time:	Cooking Time:	Servings:
15 min	60 min	4

Ingredients:

- 1½ cup beef stock
- 2 lb. pork belly
- 4 tbsp. olive oil
- Low-carb barbecue dry rub
- 2 tbsp. instant Espresso Powder.

Directions:

Set the oven at 350°F. Heat-up the beef stock in a small saucepan. Mix in the dry barbecue rub and espresso powder.

Put the pork belly, skin side up in a shallow dish and drizzle half of the oil over the top. Put the hot stock around the pork belly. Bake within 45 minutes. Sear each slice within three minutes per side. Serve.

Nutrition:

Calories: 644 kcal | Carbs: 2.6 g | Protein: 24 g | Fats: 68 g.

Garlic & Thyme Lamb Chops

Prep Time:	Cooking Time:	Servings:
15 min	10 min	6

Ingredients:

- 6 - 4 oz. lamb chops
- 4 whole garlic cloves
- 2 thyme sprigs
- 1 tsp. ground thyme
- 3 tbsp. olive oil.

Directions:

Warm-up a skillet. Put the olive oil. Rub the chops with the spices.

Put the chops in the skillet with the garlic and sprigs of thyme.

Sauté within 3 to 4 minutes and serve.

Nutrition:

Calories: 252 kcal | Carbs: 1 g | Protein: 14 g | Fats: 21 g.

Jamaican Jerk Pork Roast

Prep Time:	Cooking Time:	Servings:
15 min	4 h	12

Ingredients:

- 1 tbsp. olive oil
- 4 lb. pork shoulder
- ½ cup beef Broth
- ¼ cup Jamaican Jerk spice blend.

Directions:

Rub the roast well the oil and the jerk spice blend.

Sear the roast on all sides.

Put the beef broth.

Simmer within 4 hours on low.

Shred and serve.

Nutrition:

Calories: 282 kcal | Carbs: 0 g | Protein: 23 g | Fats: 20 g.

Keto Meatballs

Prep Time:	Cooking Time:	Servings:
15 min	20 min	10

Ingredients:

- 1 egg
- ½ cup grated parmesan
- ½ cup shredded mozzarella
- 1 lb. ground beef
- 1 tbsp. garlic.

Directions:

Warm-up the oven to reach 400°F.

Combine all of the fixings. Shape into meatballs.

Bake within 18-20 minutes.

Cool and serve.

Nutrition:

Calories: 153 kcal | Carbs: 0.7 g | Protein: 12.2 g | Fats: 10.9 g.

Mixed Vegetable Patties

Prep Time:	Cooking Time:	Servings:
15 min	10 min	4

Ingredients:

- 1 cup cauliflower florets
- 1 bag vegetables
- 1½ cup Water
- 1 cup flax meal
- 2 tbsp. olive oil.

Directions:

Steam the veggies to the steamer basket within 4 to 5 minutes.

Mash in the flax meal.

Shape into 4 patties.

Cook the patties within 3 minutes per side. Serve.

Nutrition:

Calories: 220 kcal | Carbs: 3 g | Protein: 4 g | Fats: 10 g.

Brussels Sprouts with Bacon

Prep Time:	Cooking Time:	Servings:
15 min	40 min	6

Ingredients:

- 16 oz. bacon
- 16 oz. Brussel sprouts
- Black pepper.

Directions:

Warm the oven to reach 400°F.

Slice the bacon into small lengthwise pieces. Put the sprouts and bacon with pepper.

Bake within 35 to 40 minutes. Serve.

Nutrition:

Calories: 113 kcal | Carbs: 3.9 g | Protein: 7.9 g | Total Fats: 6.9 g.

Mongolian Beef

Prep Time:	Cooking Time:	Servings:
15 min	10 min	4

Ingredients:

- 1 lb. grass-fed flank steak, cut into thin slices against the grain
- 2 tsp. arrowroot starch
- Salt, to taste
- ¼ cup avocado oil
- 1 (1-inch) piece fresh ginger, grated
- 4 garlic cloves, minced
- ½ tsp. red pepper flakes, crushed
- ¼ cup water
- ⅓ cup low-sodium soy sauce
- 1 tsp. red boat fish sauce
- 3 scallions, sliced
- 1 tsp. sesame seeds.

Direction:

In a bowl, add the steak slices, arrowroot starch, salt, and toss to coat well.

In a larger skillet, heat oil over medium-high heat and cook the steak slices for about 1½ minutes per side.

With a slotted spoon, transfer the steak slices onto a plate.

Drain the oil from the skillet but leaving about 1 tbsp. inside.

In the same skillet, add the ginger, garlic, red pepper flakes, and sauté for about 1 minute.

Add the water, soy sauce, fish sauce, and stir to combine well.

Stir in the cooked steak slices and simmer for about 3 minutes.

Stir in the scallions and simmer for about 2 minutes.

Remove from the heat and serve hot with the garnishing of sesame seeds.

Nutrition:

Calories: 266 kcal | Carbs: 5.7 g | Sugar: 1.7 g | Fiber: 1.2 g | Protein: 34 g | Fat: 11.7 g | Sodium: 1350 mg.

Chicken Schnitzel

Prep Time:	Cooking Time:	Servings:
15 min	15-22 min	4

Ingredients:

- 1 tbsp. chopped fresh parsley
- 4 garlic cloves, minced
- 1 tbsp. plain vinegar
- 1 tbsp. coconut aminos
- 2 tsp. sugar-free maple syrup
- 2 tsp. chili pepper
- Salt and black pepper to taste
- 6 tbsp. coconut oil
- 1 lb. asparagus, hard stems removed
- 4 chicken breasts, skin-on and boneless
- 2 cups grated Mexican cheese blend
- 1 tbsp. mixed sesame seeds
- 1 cup almond flour
- 4 eggs, beaten
- 6 tbsp. avocado oil
- 1 tsp. chili flakes for garnish

Directions:

In a bowl, whisk the parsley, garlic, vinegar, coconut aminos, maple syrup, chili pepper, salt, and black pepper. Set aside.

Heat the coconut oil in a large skillet and stir-fry the asparagus for 8 to 10 minutes or until tender. Remove the asparagus into a large bowl and toss with the vinegar mixture. Set aside for serving.

Cover the chicken breasts in plastic wraps and use a meat tenderizer to pound the chicken until flattened to 2-inch thickness gently.

On a plate, mix the Mexican cheese blend and sesame seeds. Dredge the chicken pieces in the almond flour, dip in the egg on both sides, and generously coat in the seed mix.

Heat the avocado oil. Cook the chicken until golden brown and cooked within.

Divide the asparagus onto four serving plates, place a chicken on each, and garnish with the chili flakes. Serve warm.

Nutrition:

Calories: 451 kcal | Fat: 18.5 g | Carbs: 5.9 g | Protein: 19.5 g.

Chicken Rollatini

Prep Time:	Cooking Time:	Servings:
15 min	30 min	4

Ingredients:

- 4 (3-ounce) boneless skinless chicken breasts, pounded to about 1/3-inch thick
- 4 oz. ricotta cheese
- 4 slices prosciutto (4 oz)
- 1 cup fresh spinach
- ½ cup almond flour
- ½ cup grated Parmesan cheese
- 2 eggs, beaten
- ¼ cup good-quality olive oil.

Directions:

Preheat the oven. Set the oven temperature to 400°F.

Prepare the chicken—Pat the chicken breasts dry with paper towels. Spread ¼ of the ricotta in the middle of each breast.

Place the prosciutto over the ricotta and ¼ cup of the spinach on the prosciutto.

Fold the long edges of the chicken breast over the filling,

then roll the chicken breast up to enclose the filling.

Place the rolls seam-side down on your work surface.

Bread the chicken. On a plate, stir together the almond flour and Parmesan and set it next to the beaten eggs.

Carefully dip a chicken roll in the egg, then roll it in the almond-flour mixture until it is completely covered.

Set the rolls seam-side down on your work surface. Repeat with the other rolls.

Brown the rolls. In a medium skillet over medium heat, warm the olive oil.

Place the rolls seam-side down in the skillet and brown them on all sides, turning them carefully, about 10 minutes in total.

Transfer the rolls, seam-side down, to a 9-by-9-inch baking dish—Bake the chicken rolls for 25 minutes, or until they're cooked through.

Serve. Place one chicken roll on each of four plates and serve them immediately.

Nutrition:

Calories: 365 kcal | Fat: 17.1 g | Fiber: 9.4 g | Carbs: 3.2 g | Protein: 1.4 g.

Roasted Leg of Lamb

Prep Time:	Cooking Time:	Servings:
15 min	1 h 30 min	6

Ingredients:

- ½ cup reduced-sodium beef broth
- 2 lb. lamb leg
- 6 garlic cloves
- 1 tbsp. rosemary leaves
- 1 tsp. black pepper.

Directions:

Warm-up oven temperature to 400°F.

Put the lamb in the pan and put the broth and seasonings.

Roast 30 minutes and lower the heat to 350°F. Cook within 1 hour.

Cool and serve.

Nutrition:

Calories: 223 kcal | Carbs: 1 g | Protein: 22 g | Fats: 14 g.

CONCLUSION

The ketogenic diet is one that has many important aspects and information that you need to know as someone who wants to try this diet. It is important to remember the warning that we have given you at the beginning of the book that this is not a diet that is safe and that doctors recommend you don't try it, or if you are going to attempt it remember that you shouldn't do so for longer than six months and even then never without the constant supervision of a doctor or at the very least a doctor knowing that you're doing this and you following their guidelines and words exactly so that they can make sure that you are safe.

The ketogenic diet is a diet that believes that by minimizing your carbs, you will while maximizing the good fat in your system and making sure that you're getting the protein you need, that you will be happier and healthier. In this book, we give you the information to know what this diet is all about, as well as describing the different types and areas that this diet will offer. Most people assume that there is only one way to do this, and while there is one thing that the additional options share, there are actually four different options you can choose from. Each one has its unique benefits, and you should know about each type to learn what would be best for your body, which is why we have described them in the book for you to have the best information possible when you begin this diet for yourself.

Another big thing about this diet is that many people don't understand the importance of exercise with this diet. The best way to become healthier is to do three things for yourself. Get the right amount of sleep, eat healthily, and make sure that you get the proper amount of exercise as well for your body to work at an optimum level. As such, we explain the exercises that are the best to go with your diet to make sure that you are getting the most out of it.

For women who are on the go and have a busy lifestyle, we have provided recipes for a thirty-day meal plan so that you can make food quickly and have a great meal for your lifestyle. They also have enough servings for you to have leftovers so that you don't have to worry about preparing in the morning. Instead, you can simply pack it up and take it with you wherever you go. This works out so much easier for so many people because they don't have to cook in the morning, and it saves a busy person a lot of time.

We also provide helpful ideas on how you can use these recipes for meals to make sure that you see how the numbers will affect you and make an impact on your day. A great example that we have explained is if you have a big breakfast that is full of the protein you need, for example, thirty g, you've got to take note of this and be aware because if you eat too much for your dinner or another meal, you will throw your numbers out of where they are supposed to be. For those that have more time on their hands, we offer a thirty-day meal plan for you as well with all-new recipes to enjoy and tips and tricks for making them work for you in the best way.

With all of this information at your fingertips, you will be able to enjoy this diet and use it to your advantage. Another benefit that we offer? We explain routines that you can do for yourself to make this diet last longer for you and to benefit your body better as a result. Routines are very important and can be a big help to your body but also your spirit and your mind. This will help you utilize the diet better, and you will be able to improve with it as well as have it become easier for you to handle.

As many people are using this diet to their benefit, knowing your food is one of the biggest parts of this, and it becomes easier once you begin to use this in your daily life. One of the best things you can do is pay attention to the food that you are eating and how it affects your body and mind. You will notice that this diet has the ability to make you sick, which isn't a good thing, and it's one of the things the doctors warn against. For this reason, it's very important to pay attention to what you are eating and how you're feeling at the same time. Another warning that we have said you need to pay attention to is that you will need to make sure that your ketogenic 'flu' isn't the result of something more serious. As people are being told that this is normal, this book has brought you the knowledge you need to be able to tell you why it's not.

This book has given you all the information you need to do this diet properly and to do it well. It's important to understand what you're getting into when you go into this diet, and this book will give you valuable information that you can use to your benefit and so you can avoid the problems that can come with this diet. You want to stay healthy and make sure that your body is able to do what it needs to. As with anything, we have put a strong emphasis on the fact that if anything feels wrong or unnatural, you will need to see a doctor to make sure that you are safe and that your body can handle this diet. Use the knowledge in this book to have amazing recipes and learn directions for amazing meals for yourself.

CPSIA information can be obtained
at www.ICGtesting.com
Printed in the USA
LVHW050027220621
690776LV00015B/1309